Healing Gemstones of the Bible

Rekishia L. McMillan, MSW
Certified Integrative Nutrition Health Coach

ISBN-13: 978-1546339953
Published by Revelation Publications

Special Note from the Author

This book is not intended to replace sound medical advice from a physician. Statements within this book have not been evaluated by the Food and Drug Administration. They are not intended to diagnose, prescribe for, treat or claim to prevent, mitigate or cure any human disease. They are intended for informational and nutritional support only. The author disclaims all liability in connection with the information presented and does not recommend, endorse or make any representation about the efficacy, appropriateness or suitability of any specific tests, products, procedures, treatments, services, opinions, health care providers or other information that may be contained on or available within this book.

You will keep in perfect peace, those whose

minds are steadfast, because they trust in

you. Trust in the Lord forever, for the Lord,

the Lord himself, is the Rock eternal.

Isaiah 26:3-4

Rock Your World Naturally

Divine Key # 2

*Love, Protect & Nurture
Your Skin*

*[Absorption / assimilate; to
take in or include as part of
oneself]*

*Do you not know that your
body is the temple of the
living God?*

I Corinthians 3:16a

What spirit is so empty and blind, that it cannot recognize the fact that the foot is more noble than the shoe, and skin more beautiful than the garment with which it is clothed?

Michelangelo

Love, Protect and Nurture Your Skin

The human body is an extraordinarily beautiful masterpiece comprised of 700 muscles, 206 bones, 30 trillion cells, and 25 miles of blood vessels and about 5 liters of blood [1].   Our internal framework of organs function in seamless fashion keeping us divinely aligned and balanced.   The human anatomy is nothing short of miraculous.   "I will praise You, for I am fearfully made; marvelous are Your works, and my soul knows very well." Psalms 139:14.

The purpose of this book is to shed light on the second of 7 Divine Keys associated with the Rock Your World Naturally Lifestyle, *"Love, Protect and Nurture Your Skin."* You'll discover why what you are putting on your skin really does matter and how wearing gemstone jewelry and using stones as a form of medicine can be beneficial to your overall health.

Skin Absorption

Often shrouded by the latest Fashionista trends, perfumes, colognes, jewelry, makeup and sprays, we rarely hear about the importance of caring for the health of the skin, but rather our focus is endlessly drawn towards the external adornment of the body. Bombarded by one new advertisement after the other, crowds are mesmerized by commercials and ads featuring a gorgeous woman, an attractive man or an adorable baby taking center stage as they showcase the latest vogue in modern makeup, designer fragrance or baby product to help keep your baby smelling "baby fresh." All the while, behind the glossy advertisements, a true endangerment to your health exists involving skin absorption.

Just How Important is Your Skin?

Although the skin is external, it is regarded as the largest organ on the human body, and covers about 20 square feet on the average size person. Along with absorption, the skin is responsible for several vital functions. Let's look at what the skin does [2].

- It holds our bodies together
- It's the first line of defense against sickness
- It serves as protective covering for the body
- It is the passage way to our bloodstream
- It helps manufacture vitamin D from the sun
- It aids in regulating our body temperature
- It aids the blood in naturally healing cuts, bruises and punctures
- Removes bodily toxins through our sweat glands

The proper care of our skin is essential to our health because skin absorbs up to 60% of what is placed on it. And the overwhelming majority of what we put on our skin includes toxic items like the jewelry we wear every day.

Toxic Jewelry and Your Health

For the most part, much attention has not been given to how wearing certain kinds of jewelry may be negatively affecting our health. Jewelry is seen as nothing more than a fashionable accessory to accent our wardrobe...rings, watches, necklaces, bracelets, earrings. They all appear to be harmless, right?   The reality of the matter is quite the contrary.

The Michigan Network for Children's Environmental Health and the Ecology Center released a study revealing that more than half, 57% of the jewelry products for children and adults tested, contained high levels of the following hazardous chemicals [3]:

- Lead

- Cadmium

- Arsenic

- Mercury

- Bromine

- Polyvinyl Chloride/Chlorine (PVC)

Studies have linked PVC in animal and some human studies to acute allergies and to long-term health impacts such as birth defects, impaired learning, liver toxicity, and cancer.

Four products contained over 10 percent cadmium, a known carcinogen. Fifty percent contained lead, with over half of these containing more than 100 ppm of lead in one or more components, exceeding the Consumer Product Safety Commission (CPSC) limit of lead in children's products [3]. Because toxic jewelry is worn regularly, these harmful substances are absorbed by the skin and directly into the blood stream, shifting the body into a dangerous state.

Skin Absorption and the Internal War

The chief function of white blood cells in the body's immune system is to protect the body against harmful substances stemming from toxins, infection, bacteria and cancerous cells. And the principal role of red blood cells is to transport oxygen to our vital organs to keep them healthy and operating at peak performance. If the blood stream is overflowing with toxins, and not cleansed regularly, how can anyone avoid contracting some form of illness? The answer is you cannot.

Barraged with toxins stemming from our everyday norms to include jewelry, food, clothing, personal care products and the environment, the blood stream becomes inundated with pollutants.

The presence of toxins causes the white blood cells into perform their role, however, too many toxins weaken and compromise the immune system. Instead of providing protection for the body, white blood cells are forced into survival mode causing confusion and malfunction within the body. The white blood cells cannot distinguish between toxins, good or bad bacteria or infections and begin attacking them all to include healthy red blood cells.

When healthy cells begin to attack themselves, this is also known as an autoimmune disorder. If this toxic cycle continues, the battle will be lost to one or more of the innumerable health disorders we see plaguing our world today in the form of arthritis, Irritable Bowel Syndrome, asthma, eczema, chronic inflammation, ADD/ADHD, psychological disorders, allergies and various cancers.

It's Time to Protect Your Skin

Your skin is the outer covering of your temple and as such, it needs proper care and attention to achieve a healthier lifestyle. We can't overlook the fact that toxins are a huge part of lives, even in the jewelry that's worn. Rest assured there are jewelry alternatives that are just as beautiful, as well as beneficial to your overall health. A good place to start is by wearing jewelry that is made from 100% pure metals, such gold, silver or copper or authentic gemstones.

Gemstones Are Part of God's Creation

Throughout the scriptures, gemstones and rocks symbolized God's strength, beauty, power and magnificence. When translated in the Old Testament, rock represented God and in the New Testament it represents Christ.

Old Testament	New Testament
1 Samuel 2:2	Matthew 7:24-27
2 Samuel 22:3	Matthew 16:18
Isaiah 17:10	Matthew 24:1
Psalms 18:2	Matthew 25:46
Psalms 28:1	Luke 8:3
Psalms 31:2-3	Romans 9:33
Psalms 89:26	1 Corinthians 10:4
Psalms 95:1	Daniel 2:45

In Exodus 28, the bible provides a clear description of the Ephod, a holy garment worn by priests that was used to know and understand the divine will of God. The Ephod was composed of fine twined linen in colors of gold, blue, purple and scarlet thread. It was beautifully crafted with 12 precious gemstones, with each stone having the name of a specific tribe inscribed on it.

The 12 Tribes and their Gemstones

1. **Ruben.** Gemstone - Sardius/Carnelian. This gem had a blood-red color, symbolic of the blood of Jesus and righteousness. In the Hebrew, it is written as Odhem and means

red.　　It was called Sardius because it was obtained from Sardis in Lydia. Exodus 28:17, 39:10 and Revelations 4:3.

2. **Simeon.**　　Gemstone - Topaz/Chrysolite. This stone is golden yellow or "green" stone brought from Cush or Ethiopia. In the Hebrew, it is written as Pitdah.　　It was the second stone in the first row in the breastplate of the high priest, and had the name of Simeon inscribed on it. Exodus 28:17, Job 28:19, Ezekiel 28:13 and 21:20.

3. **Levi.**　　Gemstone - Carbuncle/Garnet. When held up to the sun, this gem shines like a burning coal, a dark-red glowing coal. It was one of the jewels in the first row of the

high priest's breastplate. The Hebrew Ekdah is from a root meaning "to glitter," "lighten," "flash." Next to the diamond it is the hardest and most costly of all precious stones. Exodus 28:17, Exodus 39:10, Isaiah 54:12, Ezekiel 28:13Isaiah 54:12.

4. **Judah.** Gemstone - Emerald. When interpreted from the Hebrew, Nophek means the "glowing stone," and is also one of the precious stones in the breastplate of the high priest. It is mentioned Revelation 21:19 as one of the foundations of the New Jerusalem. The name given to this stone in the New Testament Greek is smaragdos, which means "live coal." Exodus 28:18, Exodus:11.

5. **Dan.** Gemstone - Sapphire. This is a precious stone of a sky-blue color brought from Babylon. It is associated with diamonds and emeralds. The throne of God is described as of the color of a sapphire. Ezekiel 28:13, 28:18, 24:10, Ezekiel 1:26).

6. **Naphtali.** Gemstone - Diamond. The Diamond, the most prized of all gemstones, is unique in several ways. It is known for being the hardest substance on earth and is sought after for its beauty and resilience. Diamonds are mentioned in the Old and New Testaments. Exodus 28:18, Exodus 39:11, Jeremiah 17:1, Ezekiel 28:13

7. **Gad.** Gemstone - Jacinth. "And the

17

foundations of the wall of the city were garnished with all manner of precious stones. The first foundation was jasper; the second, sapphire; the third, a chalcedony; the fourth, an emerald; The fifth, sardonyx; the sixth, sardius; the seventh, chrysolyte; the eighth, beryl; the ninth, a topaz; the tenth, a chrysoprasus; the eleventh, a jacinth, and the twelfth, an amethyst." Revelations 21:19-20.

8. **Asher.**   Gemstone - Agate. This stone translates in the Hebrew as Shebo, which means "ruddy," and denotes a variety of minutely crystalline silica in bands of different tints. Research shows that this stone may be the agate, a semi-transparent

crystallized quartz, probably brought from Sheba, where it derived its name. 28:19, Exodus 39:12, Isaiah 54:12 and Ezekiel 27:16.

9. **Issachar.** Gemstone - Amethyst. This stone is pale-blue crystallized quartz, varying to a dark purple blue. It is found in Persia and India and is also in different parts of Europe. Its Jewish name, was derived by the rabbis from the Hebrew word halam, meaning "to dream." Exodus 28:19, Exodus 39:12 and Revelation 21:20.

10. **Zebulun.** Gemstone - Beryl. A mineral of great hardness, and, when transparent, is extremely beautiful. When translated in

Hebrew it interprets as Tarshish. It is believed to come from Tarshish in Spain where it derives its name. The modern yellow topaz is associated with this stone. Exodus 28:20, Revelation 21:20.

11. **Joseph.** Gemstone - Onyx. There are several varieties of this stone ranging from white and reddish stripes alternating from the sardonyx; white and reddish gray, the chalcedony. In the Hebrew translation, it is Shoham meaning a nail.

12. **Benjamin.** Gemstone - Jasper. This stone is frequently mentioned throughout scripture. It was the last of the twelve stones inserted in the high priest's breastplate, and

the first of the twelve used in the foundations of the new Jerusalem. The characteristics of the stone are specified as "most precious," and "like crystal." Exodus 28:20, Exodus 39:13, Revelation 4:3, Revelation 21:11 and 21:19.

Another reference for gemstones is found in Ezekiel 28:13. Before the fall of satan, his name was Lucifer, meaning son of the morning Isaiah 14:12-15. He is described as being adorned in several precious stones:

"You were in Eden, the garden of God; every precious stone adorned you: carnelian, chrysolite and emerald, topaz, onyx and jasper, lapis lazuli, turquoise and beryl. Your settings and mountings were made of gold; on the day you were created they were prepared."

As I share in my book, *"Rock Your World Naturally: 7 Divine Keys to Unlock Extraordinary Health,"* when God created the earth, He formed it out of His Spirit, making it a spiritual entity, with everything in creation having a specific purpose.

I firmly believe that when God created gemstone they were not just intended for beauty, shelter, hunting and cooking. Much like certain forms of plant life, there are also countless species of rock that possess a wide array of healing properties that could only come from God.

In fact, century old manuscripts such as *De Materia Medica* (On Medical Material) written between 50 and 70 AD, reveal that physicians used gemstones and rock minerals alongside of plant-based treatments to help patients recover from many illnesses in the form of elixirs, pastes or alone [4]. These ancient writings are a major part of medicine and history, yet little to no modern-day scientific research has been conducted to test the validity of healing properties within gemstones.

Although not scientifically proven, why wouldn't it make sense for precious stones that were created by God to not permeate with His life-giving power?

Creation and Purpose

Without question, God is the Creator of all things. Unfortunately, over the ages, the purpose of various rocks and gemstones has been perverted and misdirected into many occult practices. This is never what God intended.   When God called the children of Israel into the promised Land of Canaan, He strongly warned them to not partake in occult practices.

"When you enter the land the Lord your God is giving you, do not learn to imitate the detestable ways of the nations there. Let no one be found among you who practices divination or sorcery, interprets omens, engages in witchcraft, or casts spells, or who is a medium or spiritist or who consults the dead. Anyone who does these things is detestable to the Lord." Deut18:9-12. And even prior to this, God made a clear distinction that He is the One true source from which ALL healing flows.

So he cried out to the LORD, and the LORD showed him a tree. When he cast it into the waters, the waters were made sweet. There He made a statute and an ordinance for them, and there He tested them, and said, "If you diligently heed the voice of the LORD your

God and do what is right in His sight, give ear to His commandments and keep all His statutes, I will put none of the diseases on you which I have brought on the Egyptians. For I am the LORD who heals you." Exodus 15:25-26.

Since the beginning of time, satan has always taken something that God has created and twisted it into a wicked practice. He does this to draw the hearts and souls of men and women away from God. My desire is for the Believer's to rethink the matter concerning His original stone creations. As Christians, our ultimate purpose is to give all glory and thanks to God for providing another avenue to bring physical healing to our bodies. You will keep in perfect peace, those whose minds are steadfast, because they trust in you. Trust in the Lord forever, for the Lord, the Lord himself, is the Rock eternal. Isaiah 26:3-4

Gemstones and Your Health

Our God is extraordinarily creative! His achievements burst with a plethora of vibrant colors. The gemstones mentioned in the bible, range from brilliant reds, oranges and yellows to calming pinks, lavender and light blues. Not only are they beautiful, they are also non-toxic when applied to the skin. This is one of the main reasons why it is so important to wear jewelry that is crafted from pure metals and/or natural gemstones. There is no need to worry about dangerous toxins being absorbed into the blood stream through the skin because gemstones are formed from natural minerals. In addition to being used for jewelry, gemstones can also be used for other health benefits. As with any healing modality, you should consult your physician prior to using any new form of treatment.

Hot Rock Therapy: Warm stones are used in this form of massage treatment to relieve tension, ease muscle stiffness and increase blood circulation and metabolism. Other ailments that can be treated are back pain, bodily aches, arthritis, osteoarthritis, stress, tension, insomnia and depression.

Cold Rock Therapy: Cold stones are an invigorating form of healing that promote blood circulation and naturally clears the body of decongestion. The use of cold stones eases inflamed tissues, reduces swelling or fluid build-up under the eyes and can also decrease muscle spasms.

Steam Rock Therapy: This form of healing is like being in a sauna. Saunas provide dry heat, while steam rock rooms use steam to induce sweating. Sweating provides numerous health benefits such as body detoxification, pain relief and improved blood circulation. Some people use steam rooms to cure different health disorders, while others use steam rock rooms to relax their body and mind.

Cancer Treatment: Diamonds are being used in various forms of cancer treatment [6]. When diamonds are released as nanodiamonds into the blood stream, medicine stays in the blood 10 times longer and has shown to be more effective.

Body Stones for Exfoliation: Pumice stones are the most widely used stones for exfoliating the skin. Exfoliating keeps the skin healthy by removing dead cells, improving circulation, opening pores to absorb moisturizers and smooths the skin.

A Call to Love the Skin You're In

While we are here on this earth, God has given us one physical body to be good and faithful stewards over. Protecting your skin is vital to your health and is based on making prayerful, educated and informed decisions. Being aware of unknown factors that silently deteriorate our health through the skin is a pre-requisite to walking in divine health. Someday, we will all shed our earthly bodies and cross over into eternity, but while we are here on earth, we can strive to live the quality of life that God has promised us by using Divine Key #2, Loving, Protecting and Nurturing the Skin that we're in.

"The foundation stones of the city wall were adorned with every kind of precious stone. The first foundation stone was; the second, sapphire; the third, chalcedony; the fourth, emerald; fifth, sardonyx; the sixth,; the seventh, chrysolite; the eighth, beryl; the ninth, topaz; the tenth, chrysoprase; the eleventh, jacinth; the twelfth, amethyst. the twelve were twelve pearls; each one of the gates was a single pearl. And the street of the city was pure gold, like transparent."

Revelations 21:19-21

ROCK YOUR WORLD NATURALLY

I pray that you were blessed by this book.

Visit my web site at

www.rockyourworldnaturally.com

and click on the book tab.

There you'll find a resource link

containing resources to help you on your

wellness journey.

What did you find most helpful?

I'd love to hear from you. E-mail me at

rockyourworldnaturally@gmail.com.

Stay Connected:

Twitter @RockYourWorld28

Facebook/RockYourWorldNaturally

Instagram/RockYourWorldNaturally

Other Books by the Author

Rock Your World Naturally:

7 Divine Keys to Unlock Extraordinary Health

References

Absorption definition -
https://www.google.com/search?q=revolution+definiti
on&rlz=1C1SNNT_enUS447&oq=revolution+definiti
on&aqs=chrome.0.0l6.3687j1j4&sourceid=chrome&e
s_sm=93&ie=UTF-8#q=absorption+definition

Unless otherwise indicated, Scripture quotations are taken from the King James Version (KJV) and New English Translation Bible public domains.

1. Phlebotomy Essentials by Ruth E. McCall, Cathee M. Tankersley, page 70.

2. Skin Problems & Treatments Health Center
http://www.webmd.com/skin-problems-and-treatments/picture-of-the-skin

3. Study on toxic jewelry
http://www.ecocenter.org/article/news-ecolink-press-releases/more-half-low-cost-jewelry-ranks-high-toxic-chemicals-new-study

4. https://en.wikipedia.org/wiki/De_Materia_Medica

5.   The Twelve Tribes and Their Gemstones. These dictionary topics are from M.G. Easton M.A., D.D., Illustrated Bible Dictionary, Third Edition, published by Thomas Nelson, 1897.   Public Domain, copy freely.

5. Onyx - Smith, William, Dr. "Entry for 'Onyx."

"Smith's Bible Dictionary".1901. and Smith, William, Dr. "Entry for 'Jasper,'". "Smith's Bible Dictionary." 1901.

6. Diamonds Healing
http://news.sciencemag.org/health/2011/03/nanodiamonds-could-be-cancer-patients-best-friend

ROCK YOUR WORLD
NATURALLY

7 DIVINE KEYS TO UNLOCK
EXTRAORDINARY HEALTH

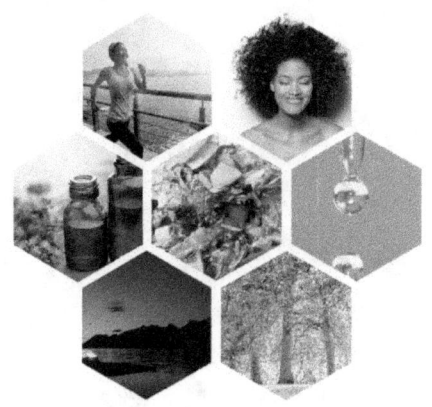

*"For the life of every living thing is in
the blood" Leviticus 17:11a*